WATER FASTING

GUIDE FOR BEGINNERS

A STEP BY STEP GUIDE TO SAFE AND EFFECTIVE FASTING

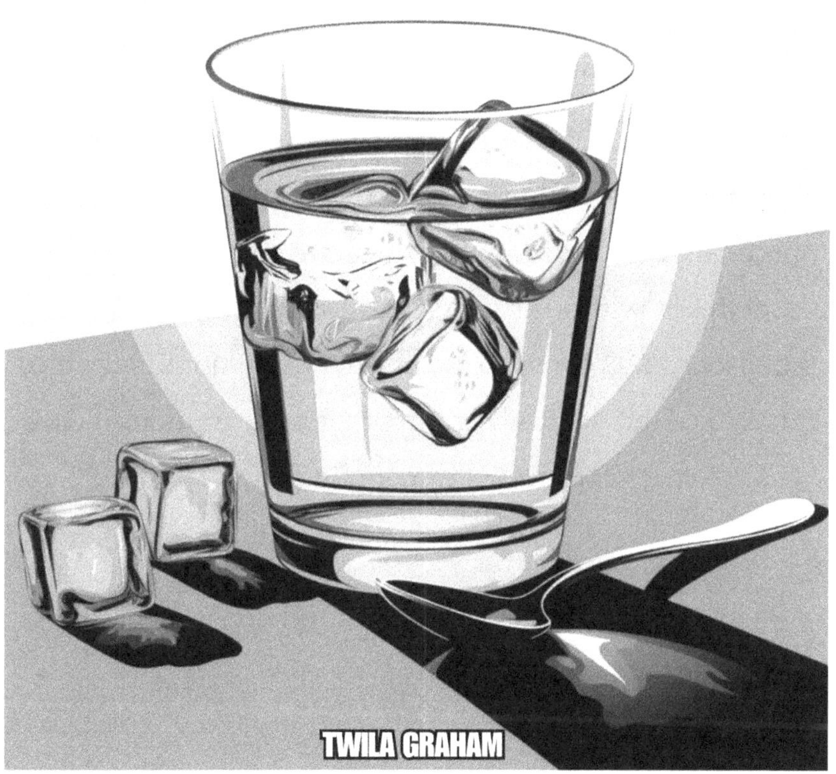

COPYRIGHT

Table of Contents

Introduction
What is Water Fasting?

DEFINITION AND OVERVIEW OF WATER FASTING

Water fasting is a type of fasting in which an individual consumes only water for a specified period, abstaining from all other food and beverages. This practice is typically done for a duration of 24 to 72 hours, though some experienced fasters may extend it longer under medical supervision. Water fasting is one of the most extreme types of fasting because it restricts all caloric intake, relying solely on the body's stored energy (in the form of glycogen and fat) to sustain metabolic processes during the fast.

Water fasting has been practiced for centuries in different cultures and religions, often for spiritual, mental, or health reasons. Today, water fasting has gained popularity as a tool for detoxifying the body, improving metabolism, promoting weight loss, and enhancing overall health.

However, it is a method that requires careful planning and medical guidance, especially for beginners or individuals with underlying health conditions.

Difference Between Water Fasting and Intermittent Fasting

Water fasting is often confused with intermittent fasting (IF), but the two are distinct in their approaches. Water fasting involves prolonged fasting periods where only water is consumed. It is generally done for several consecutive hours or days without any food intake, allowing the body to enter a deeper state of ketosis, where fat stores are broken down for energy.

Intermittent fasting, on the other hand, is a pattern of eating that alternates between periods of eating and fasting. Common forms of intermittent fasting include the 16/8 method (16 hours of fasting followed by an 8hour eating window) or the 5:2 method (eating normally for 5 days and restricting calorie intake for 2 days). While intermittent fasting focuses more on meal timing, water fasting involves complete abstinence from food, making it more challenging and intense.

HEALTH AND WELLNESS BENEFITS OF WATER FASTING

Water fasting has been linked to several potential health benefits when done safely and under supervision. These benefits include:

1. Autophagy: During prolonged fasting, the body enters a process called autophagy, where damaged or dysfunctional cells are broken down and recycled. This cellular repair mechanism can enhance longevity and reduce the risk of chronic diseases like cancer and neurodegenerative disorders.

2. Improved Insulin Sensitivity: Water fasting can help lower blood sugar levels and improve insulin sensitivity, which is beneficial for preventing or managing type 2 diabetes.

3. Weight Loss: Since no calories are consumed during water fasting, the body relies on stored fat for energy. This

can lead to significant weight loss, particularly if fasting is done regularly.

4. Detoxification: Water fasting gives the digestive system a break and allows the body to detoxify by flushing out waste products through urine and sweat. This process may leave individuals feeling lighter and more energized.

5. Mental Clarity and Focus: Many people who practice water fasting report enhanced mental clarity and focus. This may be due to the reduction of inflammation and the increased production of ketones, which fuel the brain during fasting periods.

6. Cardiovascular Health: Some studies suggest that water fasting can lower blood pressure, reduce cholesterol levels, and improve heart health by reducing inflammation and promoting better circulation.

7. Gut Health: Fasting may help reset the gut microbiome, promoting the growth of beneficial bacteria while reducing inflammation in the digestive tract.

While these benefits are promising, it is crucial to note that water fasting is not suitable for everyone. It can lead to nutrient deficiencies, dizziness, fatigue, and other health risks if not done properly. Therefore, beginners should always consult a healthcare professional before attempting a water fast to ensure it is safe for them, especially if they have existing health concerns.

UNDERSTANDING PREFASTING AND POSTFASTING MEALS

When embarking on a water fast, it's essential to consider not only the fasting period itself but also the meals consumed before and after the fast. Prefasting and postfasting meals play a critical role in preparing the body for the fasting period and helping it recover afterward.

PreFasting Meals:

Before starting a water fast, the body needs proper nourishment to prepare for the extended period without food. Prefasting meals should be light, nutrientdense, and easy to digest. These meals often include fruits, vegetables, whole grains, and lean proteins. Foods high in fiber, such as salads and soups, can also help by cleaning out the digestive system. Avoid heavy, processed, or highfat foods, as they may cause digestive discomfort and slow the transition into fasting.

PostFasting Meals:

After the fast, the body is in a sensitive state, and it's crucial to reintroduce food gradually. The first meals after fasting should be small and easy to digest to prevent overwhelming the digestive system. Start with liquids like broths, fruit juices, or smoothies, and gradually move to solid foods like vegetables, fruits, and lean proteins. Eating too much or too quickly after fasting can lead to bloating, nausea, or other gastrointestinal issues.

The right prefasting and postfasting meals will ensure that your body transitions smoothly in and out of fasting, helping you avoid adverse effects and maximize the benefits of the water fast.

IMPORTANCE OF A BALANCED APPROACH TO FASTING

While water fasting can offer significant health benefits, it is essential to approach it with balance and mindfulness. A wellbalanced fasting practice involves several factors:

Adequate hydration: During the fast, staying hydrated with plenty of water is crucial to avoid dehydration, dizziness, and fatigue. Herbal teas without sweeteners can also be included in some cases.

Preparation and refeeding: Prefasting and postfasting phases are just as important as the fasting itself. Preparing the body with nutrientrich meals and reintroducing foods slowly after fasting helps support the digestive system and prevents nutrient deficiencies.

Mindful fasting duration: For beginners, it's important not to push the body too hard. A 24hour fast is a good starting point, and longer fasts should only be attempted under medical supervision. Listen to your body and stop fasting if you experience symptoms such as dizziness, severe fatigue, or intense hunger.

Postfast recovery: After fasting, the body may need extra care. Ensure proper nutrient intake to restore energy and focus on a balanced diet to maintain the health benefits gained from fasting.

This cookbook helps provide structure and support by offering prefasting and postfasting meal ideas that are specifically designed to complement the fasting process.

How This Guide Can Help Beginners

For beginners, water fasting can seem daunting and challenging. This guide is designed to simplify the process, offering stepbystep instructions, meal ideas, and valuable insights to ensure a safe and effective fasting experience.

Clear instructions: The cookbook breaks down the fasting process into manageable stages, starting with how to prepare the body before the fast, guidance during the fast itself, and tips for refeeding after the fast.

Meal suggestions: The guide includes nutritious, easytodigest recipes that are tailored to each phase of fasting. These recipes are designed to help beginners nourish their bodies before and after the fast, promoting a smooth and healthy fasting experience.

Nutritional balance: For those new to fasting, the cookbook emphasizes the importance of maintaining a balanced diet outside of the fasting window. It provides nutrientdense, whole food recipes that are rich in vitamins, minerals, and essential nutrients, ensuring that beginners do not compromise their health during the fasting process.

Expert tips: With practical tips and advice throughout the guide, beginners will learn how to listen to their bodies, avoid common pitfalls, and make the most of the fasting experience. The guide also offers suggestions for different fasting lengths and explains when to seek medical advice.

This Water Fasting Cookbook is designed to take the guesswork out of fasting, offering a comprehensive, beginnerfriendly resource that empowers individuals to fast safely and successfully.

Chapter 1

Mental and Emotional Preparation

Setting Realistic Expectations

Before beginning a water fast, one of the most important steps is setting realistic expectations. This involves understanding the physical, mental, and emotional challenges that come with fasting. Many beginners may assume that fasting is simply abstaining from food, but the process is much more complex. The body undergoes several changes, such as shifts in metabolism, hormone regulation, and energy levels. By setting realistic expectations, you can better prepare for these changes and minimize potential frustration or disappointment.

Fasting for extended periods can lead to common symptoms like headaches, dizziness, fatigue, and irritability, especially in the early stages. Understanding that these are normal responses will help you remain patient and continue the fast. It's crucial to recognize that water fasting is not a quick fix, but rather a gradual process that requires discipline, awareness, and time to see the full benefits.

When setting expectations, consider the following:

Duration of the fast: Beginners should start with shorter fasts, such as 24 hours, before attempting longer ones. This allows the body to adjust gradually and helps you understand how fasting affects you personally.

Weight loss and other health benefits: While many people water fast to lose weight, the process is not instantaneous. The initial drop in weight often comes from water loss, and longterm results require consistency and proper refeeding afterward.

Mental clarity: Many fasters experience mental clarity after a certain period of fasting, but this usually occurs after overcoming initial physical discomforts. Knowing this in advance can help keep you motivated.

Realistic expectations reduce the likelihood of feeling overwhelmed or discouraged. It's important to have a clear purpose and to pace yourself, focusing on progress rather than perfection.

Building a Mindset for Success and Discipline

Mental and emotional preparation is equally critical to physical readiness when starting a water fast. Developing a mindset geared toward success and discipline will help you stay committed, even when the fast becomes challenging.

Fasting requires mental strength because hunger, cravings, and fatigue can cause moments of doubt or desire to quit. A successful fast begins with setting clear intentions and understanding why you're fasting. Whether your goal is weight loss, detoxification, spiritual growth, or mental clarity, having a solid "why" will serve as a foundation for discipline.

Key components for building a fasting mindset include:

Visualization and affirmation: Visualizing the results you want to achieve can reinforce your determination during difficult moments. Affirmations such as "I am in control of my body," or "I am strong enough to complete this fast," can also be powerful tools for maintaining mental focus.

Patience and selfcompassion: Fasting can test your patience, especially during the first few days when cravings and discomfort peak. Being kind to yourself and understanding that each stage of the fast brings new challenges can help you persevere. Instead of being hard on yourself for feeling hungry or tired, acknowledge these feelings and remind yourself of the temporary nature of discomfort.

Managing emotions: Fasting can bring emotional changes. Some individuals experience mood swings or feel emotionally vulnerable, especially as they confront the relationship between food and comfort. Taking time to reflect on your emotional connection with food can offer valuable insights into personal habits. Journaling or meditating during your fast can help you process these emotions and maintain mental clarity.

Support and accountability: For many people, having a support system during fasting can make a big difference. Whether it's a fasting community, a friend who's done fasting before, or an online group, sharing your journey can offer emotional support and motivation. If you're fasting alone, keeping a journal of your experience can serve as a form of selfaccountability.

In summary, fasting is as much a mental and emotional process as it is a physical one. Approaching it with the right mindset—where patience, discipline, and selfawareness are key—ensures a smoother, more successful fasting experience. By mentally preparing yourself, you'll have the emotional resilience needed to overcome obstacles, making your fasting journey more rewarding in the end.

The Importance of PreFast Nutrition

Proper dietary preparation is essential before starting a water fast. How you prepare your body in the days leading up to the fast can significantly affect how smoothly the fast goes, as well as the benefits you experience. Pre Fast nutrition ensures that your body is nourished, energized, and ready to handle the absence of food for the fasting period. It helps minimize the intensity of common fasting side effects, such as headaches, fatigue, and irritability, by stabilizing blood sugar levels and balancing electrolytes beforehand.

When the body is well prepared through prefast nutrition, the transition into the fast is smoother, and it can more easily adapt to using fat stores for energy instead of relying on glucose from recent meals. Proper prefasting nutrition also helps reduce food cravings and hunger pangs, making it mentally easier to adhere to the fasting period. Hydration during this time is equally important, as entering a water fast while dehydrated can lead to more pronounced symptoms of dizziness and weakness.

RECOMMENDED FOODS TO EAT BEFORE A WATER FAST

Leading up to your water fast, it's important to gradually reduce your calorie intake while focusing on nutrientdense foods that prepare your body for the upcoming fasting period. This gradual reduction allows your digestive system to slow down, helping you avoid sudden hunger pangs or cravings when you begin the fast.

Key foods to incorporate before fasting include:

Fruits and Vegetables: These are rich in fiber, vitamins, and antioxidants, which help cleanse the digestive system. Opt for light, waterrich fruits like cucumbers, melons, and citrus fruits, as well as leafy greens like spinach, kale, and romaine lettuce.

Whole Grains: Brown rice, quinoa, oats, and barley can be consumed in moderate portions to provide slowreleasing carbohydrates. These grains help stabilize blood sugar levels, preventing drastic energy drops early in the fast.

Lean Proteins: Include small amounts of lean protein sources such as chicken breast, turkey, and fish in the days before fasting. These proteins are easier to digest and help maintain muscle mass without overloading the digestive system.

Healthy Fats: Avocados, nuts, seeds, and olive oil are great sources of healthy fats that promote satiety and nourish the body. These fats provide a longerlasting energy source and help your body adjust to the switch to fatburning during fasting.

Hydrating Foods and Fluids: Drink plenty of water, herbal teas, and consume waterdense foods like watermelon and cucumbers to maintain hydration. Coconut water is a great prefasting beverage as it replenishes electrolytes.

To make the transition to fasting easier, it's advisable to eat smaller, lighter meals for a few days leading up to the fast. A common approach is to progressively reduce meal sizes while increasing the intake of fluids and hydrating foods.

Foods to Avoid Before Fasting

Certain foods should be avoided before starting a water fast, as they can lead to blood sugar spikes, cravings, digestive discomfort, and even hinder the benefits of fasting.

Avoiding these foods will allow your body to enter the fasting state more smoothly, and reduce the intensity of any negative symptoms during the fast.

Sugary Foods: Highsugar foods such as candy, cakes, cookies, and sugary beverages cause sharp increases in blood sugar levels followed by rapid crashes. These fluctuations can make the initial phase of fasting more difficult as the body craves more sugar.

Processed and Packaged Foods: Processed foods are typically high in refined carbohydrates, preservatives, and unhealthy fats. These foods are harder for the body to digest and can lead to bloating or discomfort at the start of a fast. Examples include chips, fast food, frozen meals, and anything high in artificial additives.

Caffeine and Alcohol: Both caffeine and alcohol are dehydrating and can disrupt the body's natural hydration levels. Caffeine can also cause spikes in energy followed by sudden drops, which can increase feelings of fatigue during fasting. Similarly, alcohol consumption can lead to dehydration and interfere with liver detoxification, making fasting more taxing on the body.

Dairy and Heavy Animal Proteins: Foods like red meat, cheese, and creamy dishes are slow to digest and can place a heavy burden on the digestive system. Eating these foods right before a fast can make the transition harder on the body as it shifts to ketosis.

By gradually reducing your intake of these foods and focusing on light, nutrientdense options, you can ensure that your body is wellprepared for the water fast ahead. This preparation phase sets the foundation for a smoother fasting experience and helps maximize the benefits of the fast..

HOW MUCH WATER TO DRINK DURING A FAST

Hydration is the cornerstone of a successful water fast, as your body depends on water for nearly every function. During a water fast, it's important to maintain proper hydration levels since no other fluids or foods are consumed. A general recommendation is to drink 2 to 3 liters of water per day, but this amount can vary based on individual factors such as body weight, activity levels, climate, and health conditions.

It's essential to spread out your water intake throughout the day rather than drinking large amounts all at once. This helps your body better absorb the water and maintain hydration without overwhelming the kidneys. Thirst is a natural indicator, but it's important to be proactive about hydration, especially during the first few days of fasting, as dehydration can occur without the usual cues of eating or drinking.

Sipping water slowly throughout the day is more effective than drinking large quantities in one sitting, which can cause an imbalance in electrolytes and potentially lead to symptoms like headaches, dizziness, or nausea. You may also adjust your water intake based on activity; if you're physically active, you may need to drink more to compensate for the fluids lost through sweat. In cooler climates or lower activity levels, a slightly lower intake may suffice.

To stay adequately hydrated, it is helpful to set reminders to drink water regularly. Using a water bottle with markers that show how much you've consumed by certain times of the day can also assist in keeping track.

ELECTROLYTE CONSIDERATIONS AND HYDRATION TIPS

While water is vital for hydration, electrolytes — minerals like sodium, potassium, magnesium, and calcium — are just as important for maintaining the balance of fluids in your body. During prolonged water fasting, the body naturally flushes out electrolytes, which can result in an imbalance, causing symptoms like dizziness, fatigue, muscle cramps, and even confusion. Ensuring proper electrolyte intake is crucial for avoiding these adverse effects.

Though traditional water fasting does not include the intake of supplements or any food, some modified fasting approaches allow for the inclusion of small amounts of electrolytes to maintain health. This can be done through adding a pinch of sea salt to your water, consuming diluted mineral water, or using electrolyte supplements designed specifically for fasting.

To further improve hydration, consider these additional tips:

Room Temperature or Warm Water: Drinking water at room temperature or slightly warm is gentler on the stomach and easier for the body to absorb. Cold water can sometimes cause digestive discomfort or increase thirst.

Herbal Teas: If permitted in your fasting protocol, unsweetened herbal teas can be a good way to increase fluid intake. Peppermint, chamomile, or ginger teas can also help with nausea or upset stomachs.

Avoid Carbonated or Flavored Waters: While tempting, carbonated or artificially flavored waters can create bloating, gas, or discomfort during fasting. Stick to plain water or natural mineral water.

FASTING SAFETY AND PRECAUTIONS

Who Should Consult a Doctor Before Fasting

Though water fasting offers numerous health benefits, it's not suitable for everyone, and certain individuals should consult a doctor before attempting a water fast. Medical supervision is especially important for people with preexisting health conditions, as fasting can exacerbate certain medical issues or interfere with medications.

Individuals with Chronic Conditions: Those with diabetes, high blood pressure, heart disease, kidney disease, or any chronic illness should seek medical advice before fasting. For example, water fasting can lead to drastic blood sugar changes, which may be dangerous for individuals with diabetes. Kidney function can also be compromised, particularly for those who already have kidney problems, as the body's need to filter and balance electrolytes increases during fasting.

Pregnant or Breastfeeding Women: Fasting is not recommended for pregnant or breastfeeding women because it may deprive both the mother and child of necessary nutrients. Adequate calorie and nutrient intake are critical for supporting fetal development and milk production.

Individuals with Eating Disorders: Those with a history of eating disorders like anorexia, bulimia, or binge eating should avoid fasting. Fasting can trigger unhealthy behaviors or psychological distress, which can lead to a relapse in disordered eating patterns.

Underweight Individuals: Those who are already underweight or malnourished should avoid water fasting, as it can further exacerbate nutritional deficiencies and cause unhealthy weight loss.

People Taking Medications: Certain medications, such as blood thinners, heart medications, and antiseizure drugs, can interact with fasting. The absence of food can alter how medications are absorbed, potentially leading to side effects or reduced efficacy.

A healthcare provider can offer personalized advice and may recommend a modified fasting approach or intermittent fasting as a safer alternative.

Fasting Red Flags: When to Stop

Fasting should always be approached with caution, and it's important to know the signs that indicate you should stop fasting immediately. While mild symptoms like headaches, fatigue, and irritability are common during the first few days of fasting, more severe symptoms can signal that your body is in distress.

Red flags that indicate you should stop fasting include:

Severe Dizziness or Fainting: Feeling lightheaded or fainting is a serious sign that your body may not be getting enough energy or fluids. If you experience extreme dizziness or lose consciousness, stop the fast and seek medical help.

Confusion or Disorientation: Mental fog or mild confusion can be a normal part of fasting for some individuals, but severe disorientation, memory loss, or trouble concentrating are red flags. These symptoms may indicate dangerously low blood sugar or electrolyte imbalances.

Heart Palpitations: If you notice an irregular heartbeat or feel your heart racing, this can indicate an electrolyte imbalance or dehydration. Palpitations are a sign that your heart is working harder than normal, and the body may not have enough minerals to support proper function.

Severe Weakness or Fatigue: While mild fatigue is normal, extreme weakness or an inability to perform basic tasks is not. If you find yourself unable to walk, stand up, or move around easily, it's time to end the fast.

Persistent Nausea or Vomiting: Feeling nauseous during a fast can be a sign that your digestive system is struggling to adjust, but if nausea becomes persistent or you start vomiting, it's essential to stop the fast. Vomiting can lead to dehydration and disrupt electrolyte balance.

Abdominal Pain or Cramping: Mild digestive discomfort is normal during fasting, but severe abdominal pain, cramping, or bloating may indicate an underlying issue that needs attention.

If you experience any of these symptoms, it's crucial to break the fast safely by consuming small, nutrientdense foods and hydrating with electrolyterich fluids. Continuing to fast despite these warning signs can lead to serious health complications. Always listen to your body and err on the side of caution when it comes to fasting.

Chapter 5

NutrientRich Soups and Broths (10 Recipes)

VEGETABLE BROTH FOR REFEEDING

Light, LowSodium Vegetable Broth

Servings: 4

Prep Time: 10 minutes

Cook Time: 45 minutes

Ingredients:

4 cups filtered water

2 carrots, peeled and chopped

2 celery stalks, chopped

1 onion, peeled and quartered

1 small zucchini, chopped

2 garlic cloves, smashed

1 bay leaf

Fresh parsley, a small bunch

½ tsp ground turmeric (optional)

½ tsp sea salt (optional)

Instructions:

1. In a large pot, combine all the vegetables and water.

2. Bring to a boil, then reduce heat to simmer for 45 minutes.

3. Strain the broth through a fine mesh sieve to remove the solids.

4. Season with sea salt (optional) and serve warm. This light broth is ideal for reintroducing nutrients postfast.

Nutritional Information (per serving):

Calories: 35 kcal

Protein: 1 g

Fat: 0 g

Carbohydrates: 8 g

Sodium: 40 mg

Bone Broth for Healing

NutrientDense Chicken Bone Broth with Herbs

Servings: 6

Prep Time: 15 minutes

Cook Time: 68 hours

Ingredients:

1 whole chicken carcass (organic)

8 cups water

2 carrots, roughly chopped

2 celery stalks, roughly chopped

1 onion, quartered

2 garlic cloves, smashed

1 tbsp apple cider vinegar

1 bay leaf

Fresh thyme or rosemary (optional)

Sea salt and pepper to taste

Instructions:

1. Place the chicken carcass in a large stockpot or slow cooker.

2. Add water, apple cider vinegar, and vegetables. Let it sit for 10 minutes.

3. Bring the broth to a gentle simmer and cook on low heat for 68 hours.

4. Skim off any foam that rises to the surface and discard.

5. Strain the broth through a sieve, discarding solids. Season with salt and pepper.

6. Allow the broth to cool before serving or refrigerating.

Nutritional Information (per serving):

Calories: 85 kcal

Protein: 7 g

Fat: 5 g

Carbohydrates: 4 g

Sodium: 100 mg

These recipes serve as nutrientrich foundations to refeed and restore the body after fasting, promoting digestion and hydration.

NOURISHING SOUPS

Miso Soup with Seaweed and Tofu

Servings: 4

Prep Time: 10 minutes

Cook Time: 15 minutes

Ingredients:

4 cups water

2 tbsp miso paste (white or yellow)

1 cup tofu, cubed

1 cup dried seaweed (wakame), rehydrated

2 green onions, thinly sliced

1 small piece of ginger, peeled and sliced

1 garlic clove, minced (optional)

1 tbsp soy sauce (optional)

Instructions:

1. In a pot, bring water to a boil and add ginger and garlic (if using). Simmer for 5 minutes.

2. Dissolve the miso paste in a small amount of hot water and stir into the pot.

3. Add tofu and rehydrated seaweed. Simmer for 5 minutes, ensuring the tofu is heated through.

4. Stir in green onions and soy sauce (if using). Serve hot.

Nutritional Information (per serving):

Calories: 80 kcal

Protein: 7 g

Fat: 4 g

Carbohydrates: 6 g

Sodium: 800 mg

Carrot Ginger Soup with Coconut Milk

Servings: 4

Prep Time: 15 minutes

Cook Time: 30 minutes

Ingredients:

4 cups vegetable broth

1 lb carrots, peeled and chopped

1 onion, chopped

2 tbsp fresh ginger, grated

1 can (13.5 oz) coconut milk

2 tbsp olive oil

1 tsp ground cumin

Salt and pepper to taste

Instructions:

1. Heat olive oil in a pot over medium heat. Add onions and ginger, cooking until fragrant (about 5 minutes).

2. Add carrots, cumin, and vegetable broth. Bring to a boil, then reduce heat and simmer until carrots are tender (20 minutes).

3. Use an immersion blender to puree the soup until smooth. Stir in coconut milk.

4. Season with salt and pepper to taste. Serve warm.

Nutritional Information (per serving):

Calories: 190 kcal

Protein: 2 g

Fat: 13 g

Carbohydrates: 17 g

Sodium: 300 mg

DETOXIFYING SOUP

Green Detox Soup with Spinach, Kale, and Broccoli

Servings: 4

Prep Time: 15 minutes

Cook Time: 30 minutes

Ingredients:

4 cups vegetable broth

1 cup broccoli florets

2 cups spinach

2 cups kale, stems removed and chopped

1 onion, chopped

2 garlic cloves, minced

1 zucchini, chopped

1 tbsp olive oil

1 tsp dried thyme

Salt and pepper to taste

Instructions:

1. Heat olive oil in a large pot over medium heat. Add onions and garlic, cooking until softened (5 minutes).

2. Add zucchini and cook for another 5 minutes.

3. Pour in vegetable broth and bring to a boil. Reduce heat and add broccoli. Simmer until broccoli is tender (10 minutes).

4. Add spinach and kale. Cook for an additional 5 minutes until greens are wilted.

5. Use an immersion blender to puree the soup until smooth. Season with salt, pepper, and thyme. Serve hot.

Nutritional Information (per serving):

Calories: 110 kcal

Protein: 5 g

Fat: 4 g

Carbohydrates: 15 g

Sodium: 400 mg

These recipes are designed to provide essential nutrients while supporting the body's natural detoxification processes. They are light yet nourishing, ideal for those breaking a fast or seeking a nutrient boost.

Chapter 6

Light, EasytoDigest Meals (10 Recipes)

VegetableBased Meals

Zucchini Noodles with Light Pesto

Servings: 4

Prep Time: 15 minutes

Cook Time: 10 minutes

Ingredients:

4 medium zucchinis, spiralized into noodles

1 cup fresh basil leaves

2 tbsp pine nuts (or walnuts)

2 cloves garlic

¼ cup extravirgin olive oil

¼ cup grated Parmesan cheese (optional)

Salt and pepper to taste

Instructions:

1. In a food processor, combine basil, pine nuts, garlic, and olive oil. Blend until smooth, adding more oil if needed.

2. Heat a large skillet over medium heat. Add zucchini noodles and sauté for 23 minutes until slightly tender.

3. Toss the zucchini noodles with the pesto sauce. If using, sprinkle with Parmesan cheese and season with salt and pepper.

4. Serve immediately.

Nutritional Information (per serving):

Calories: 200 kcal

Protein: 5 g

Fat: 16 g

Carbohydrates: 12 g

Sodium: 150 mg

Roasted Butternut Squash with Quinoa

Servings: 4

Prep Time: 10 minutes

Cook Time: 30 minutes

Ingredients:

1 medium butternut squash, peeled and cubed

2 tbsp olive oil

1 tsp ground cumin

1 tsp paprika

1 cup quinoa

2 cups vegetable broth

2 tbsp fresh parsley, chopped

Salt and pepper to taste

Instructions:

1. Preheat oven to 400°F (200°C). Toss butternut squash cubes with olive oil, cumin, paprika, salt, and pepper. Spread on a baking sheet.

2. Roast for 2530 minutes, until tender and slightly caramelized.

3. While the squash is roasting, rinse quinoa under cold water. In a pot, combine quinoa and vegetable broth. Bring to a boil, then reduce heat to simmer. Cook for 15 minutes or until quinoa is tender and liquid is absorbed.

4. Fluff quinoa with a fork and mix in roasted butternut squash. Garnish with fresh parsley.

Nutritional Information (per serving):

Calories: 250 kcal

Protein: 8 g

Fat: 10 g

Carbohydrates: 35 g

Sodium: 200 mg

These recipes focus on vegetables and whole grains, providing light, nutrientdense meals that are easy to digest and perfect for maintaining a balanced diet during or after a water fast.

ProteinRich Light Dishes

Soft Boiled Eggs with Asparagus

Servings: 2

Prep Time: 10 minutes

Cook Time: 10 minutes

Ingredients:

4 large eggs

1 bunch asparagus, trimmed

1 tbsp olive oil

1 lemon, zest and juice

Salt and pepper to taste

Instructions:

1. Bring a pot of water to a boil. Carefully add eggs and cook for 67 minutes for softboiled. Transfer eggs to an ice bath to cool.

2. While the eggs are cooking, heat olive oil in a skillet over medium heat. Add asparagus and cook for 45 minutes until tendercrisp.

3. Season asparagus with salt, pepper, and lemon zest. Toss to coat.

4. Peel the eggs and halve them. Serve alongside the asparagus with a squeeze of lemon juice.

Nutritional Information (per serving):

Calories: 240 kcal

Protein: 14 g

Fat: 16 g

Carbohydrates: 8 g

Sodium: 180 mg

BAKED COD WITH STEAMED CARROTS

Servings: 2

Prep Time: 10 minutes

Cook Time: 20 minutes

Ingredients:

2 cod fillets (6 oz each)

1 tbsp olive oil

1 lemon, sliced

1 tsp dried thyme

1 tsp garlic powder

1 bunch carrots, peeled and cut into sticks

Salt and pepper to taste

Instructions:

1. Preheat oven to 375°F (190°C). Place cod fillets on a baking sheet lined with parchment paper. Drizzle with olive oil and season with thyme, garlic powder, salt, and pepper. Top with lemon slices.

2. Bake for 1520 minutes, until cod flakes easily with a fork.

3. Meanwhile, steam carrot sticks in a steamer basket over boiling water for about 8 minutes, or until tender.

4. Serve the baked cod with steamed carrots on the side.

Nutritional Information (per serving):

Calories: 290 kcal

Protein: 28 g

Fat: 12 g

Carbohydrates: 14 g

Sodium: 210 mg

These proteinrich light dishes provide a balanced approach to easytodigest meals, offering both highquality protein and essential nutrients in a gentle, easily assimilated format.

POSTFAST VEGAN OPTIONS

Lentil and Sweet Potato Stew

Servings: 4

Prep Time: 15 minutes

Cook Time: 35 minutes

Ingredients:

1 cup dried green or brown lentils, rinsed

1 medium sweet potato, peeled and diced

1 onion, chopped

2 cloves garlic, minced

2 carrots, diced

1 celery stalk, diced

1 can diced tomatoes (14.5 oz)

4 cups vegetable broth

1 tsp ground cumin

1 tsp smoked paprika

1/2 tsp turmeric

2 tbsp olive oil

Salt and pepper to taste

2 cups fresh spinach

Instructions:

1. Heat olive oil in a large pot over medium heat. Add onion, garlic, carrots, and celery. Sauté for 57 minutes until vegetables are softened.

2. Stir in the cumin, smoked paprika, and turmeric. Cook for 1 minute until fragrant.

3. Add lentils, sweet potato, diced tomatoes, and vegetable broth. Bring to a boil, then reduce heat to low. Simmer for 2530 minutes, until lentils and sweet potato are tender.

4. Stir in fresh spinach and cook for an additional 2 minutes until wilted. Season with salt and pepper to taste.

5. Serve hot.

Nutritional Information (per serving):

Calories: 280 kcal

Protein: 13 g

Fat: 8 g

Carbohydrates: 41 g

Sodium: 500 mg

Grilled Portobello Mushrooms with Spinach

Servings: 4

Prep Time: 10 minutes

Cook Time: 15 minutes

Ingredients:

4 large Portobello mushroom caps

2 tbsp balsamic vinegar

2 tbsp olive oil

2 cloves garlic, minced

1 tsp dried oregano

1 tsp dried basil

Salt and pepper to taste

2 cups fresh spinach

1 tbsp lemon juice

Instructions:

1. Preheat grill to mediumhigh heat. In a small bowl, mix balsamic vinegar, olive oil, garlic, oregano, basil, salt, and pepper.

2. Brush the Portobello mushrooms with the balsamic mixture. Grill mushrooms for 45 minutes per side, until tender and slightly charred.

3. While the mushrooms are grilling, heat a large skillet over medium heat. Add spinach and sauté until wilted, about 2 minutes. Toss with lemon juice.

4. Serve grilled mushrooms on a bed of sautéed spinach.

Nutritional Information (per serving):

Calories: 180 kcal

Protein: 5 g

Fat: 14 g

Carbohydrates: 13 g

Sodium: 200 mg

These postfast vegan options are designed to gently reintroduce nutrients and energy into your diet while remaining easy to digest and nourishing.

Chapter 7

Smoothies and Juices for Pre and PostFast (10 Recipes)

HYDRATING PREFAST SMOOTHIES

Coconut Water Smoothie with Pineapple and Chia Seeds

Servings: 2

Prep Time: 5 minutes

Ingredients:

1 cup coconut water

1 cup fresh pineapple chunks

1 tbsp chia seeds

1 banana

1/2 cup Greek yogurt (optional for creaminess)

Ice cubes (optional)

Instructions:

1. In a blender, combine coconut water, pineapple chunks, chia seeds, banana, and Greek yogurt (if using).

2. Blend until smooth. Add ice cubes if desired and blend again until frothy.

3. Pour into glasses and serve immediately.

Nutritional Information (per serving):

Calories: 190 kcal

Protein: 4 g

Fat: 4 g

Carbohydrates: 38 g

Sodium: 50 mg

SPINACH, APPLE, AND GINGER DETOX JUICE

Servings: 2

Prep Time: 10 minutes

Ingredients:

2 cups fresh spinach leaves

2 medium apples, cored and sliced

1inch piece of fresh ginger, peeled

1/2 lemon, juiced

1 cup water or coconut water

Instructions:

1. Juice the spinach, apples, and ginger in a juicer.

2. Add lemon juice and water (or coconut water) to the juice.

3. Stir well and serve chilled.

Nutritional Information (per serving):

Calories: 120 kcal

Protein: 2 g

Fat: 0 g

Carbohydrates: 30 g

Sodium: 10 mg

These hydrating smoothies are perfect for preparing your body for a water fast, providing essential nutrients and hydration while being light and easy on the digestive system.

POSTFAST SMOOTHIES

Banana and Almond Milk Smoothie

Servings: 2

Prep Time: 5 minutes

Ingredients:

2 ripe bananas

1 cup unsweetened almond milk

1 tbsp almond butter

1 tbsp honey or maple syrup (optional for sweetness)

1/2 tsp vanilla extract

Ice cubes (optional)

Instructions:

1. In a blender, combine bananas, almond milk, almond butter, honey (if using), and vanilla extract.

2. Blend until smooth. Add ice cubes if desired and blend again until frothy.

3. Pour into glasses and serve immediately.

Nutritional Information (per serving):

Calories: 220 kcal

Protein: 4 g

Fat: 9 g

Carbohydrates: 32 g

Sodium: 150 mg

WATERMELON AND CUCUMBER HYDRATING JUICE

Servings: 2

Prep Time: 10 minutes

Ingredients:

2 cups cubed watermelon

1 cup cucumber, peeled and chopped

1/2 lime, juiced

1 tbsp fresh mint leaves (optional)

1 cup cold water

Instructions:

1. In a blender, combine watermelon, cucumber, and lime juice. Blend until smooth.

2. Strain the mixture through a fine mesh sieve or cheesecloth if desired for a smoother texture.

3. Stir in fresh mint leaves if using. Serve chilled.

Nutritional Information (per serving):

Calories: 90 kcal

Protein: 1 g

Fat: 0 g

Carbohydrates: 23 g

Sodium: 10 mg

These postfast smoothies and juices are designed to gently reintroduce flavors and nutrients while being easy on the digestive system, helping to restore energy and hydration.

ELECTROLYTERICH DRINKS

Lemon Coconut Water Refresher

Servings: 2

Prep Time: 5 minutes

Ingredients:

2 cups coconut water

Juice of 1 lemon

12 tbsp honey or maple syrup (optional, for sweetness)

1/4 tsp sea salt

Fresh mint leaves for garnish (optional)

Instructions:

1. In a pitcher, combine coconut water and lemon juice.

2. Stir in honey or maple syrup if using, and sea salt. Mix until the sweetener and salt are fully dissolved.

3. Pour the mixture over ice in glasses.

4. Garnish with fresh mint leaves if desired, and serve immediately.

Nutritional Information (per serving):

Calories: 80 kcal

Protein: 0 g

Fat: 0 g

Carbohydrates: 20 g

Sodium: 190 mg

Explanation:

Coconut water is a natural source of electrolytes like potassium, sodium, and magnesium, making it an excellent choice for replenishing electrolytes lost during fasting. The addition of lemon juice enhances the drink with a dose of vitamin C and provides a refreshing, tangy flavor. Honey or maple syrup adds a touch of natural sweetness, while sea salt helps replace sodium and balance electrolytes. This drink is designed to hydrate and restore essential minerals, supporting overall electrolyte balance and aiding recovery postfast.

Cucumber Mint Juice with Electrolytes

Servings: 2

Prep Time: 10 minutes

Ingredients:

1 large cucumber, peeled and chopped

Juice of 1 lime

1/2 cup coconut water

1 tbsp chia seeds (optional, for added hydration and nutrients)

A few fresh mint leaves

12 tbsp honey or agave syrup (optional, for sweetness)

Instructions:

1. In a blender, combine cucumber, lime juice, and coconut water. Blend until smooth.

2. Strain the mixture through a fine mesh sieve or cheesecloth to remove pulp if desired.

3. Stir in chia seeds if using and let the mixture sit for a few minutes to allow the seeds to expand.

4. Sweeten with honey or agave syrup if desired, and garnish with fresh mint leaves.

5. Serve chilled.

Nutritional Information (per serving):

Calories: 70 kcal

Protein: 1 g

Fat: 0 g

Carbohydrates: 16 g

Sodium: 30 mg

Explanation:

Cucumber is incredibly hydrating and contains electrolytes like potassium, which help maintain fluid balance in the body. Lime juice adds a zesty flavor and boosts vitamin C content. Coconut water provides additional electrolytes, enhancing the drink's effectiveness in replenishing lost minerals. Chia seeds, if added, contribute omega3 fatty acids and fiber, further supporting hydration and digestive health. This juice is designed to be both refreshing and effective in restoring electrolytes, making it an ideal choice for recovery after fasting or intense physical activity.

These electrolyterich drinks are crafted to assist in hydration and mineral replenishment, crucial for maintaining balance and supporting overall wellbeing during and after a water fast.

Chapter 8

Healing and Restorative Foods PostFasting (10 Recipes)

FERMENTED FOODS FOR GUT HEALTH

Sauerkraut and Kimchi with Avocado

Servings: 2

Prep Time: 10 minutes

Ingredients:

1 cup sauerkraut, drained

1 cup kimchi, drained

1 ripe avocado, sliced

1 tbsp sesame seeds

1 tbsp chopped fresh cilantro (optional)

1 tbsp extra virgin olive oil (optional)

Salt and pepper to taste

Instructions:

1. In a bowl, combine sauerkraut and kimchi. Mix well.

2. Arrange the avocado slices on plates or in bowls.

3. Top with the sauerkraut and kimchi mixture.

4. Sprinkle with sesame seeds and chopped cilantro if using.

5. Drizzle with olive oil if desired, and season with salt and pepper.

6. Serve immediately.

Nutritional Information (per serving):

Calories: 150 kcal

Protein: 3 g

Fat: 9 g

Carbohydrates: 15 g

Sodium: 800 mg

Explanation:

Sauerkraut and kimchi are both rich in probiotics, which are beneficial bacteria that help restore gut flora balance. The fermentation process enhances the nutritional content of these foods, making them excellent for supporting digestion and gut health. Avocado adds healthy fats and fiber, which can aid in digestion and provide a creamy texture that complements the tanginess of the fermented vegetables. This combination supports overall gut health and helps ease the transition back to regular eating postfast.

ProbioticRich Meals

Greek Yogurt with Honey and Blueberries

Servings: 2

Prep Time: 5 minutes

Ingredients:

1 cup plain Greek yogurt

1/4 cup fresh blueberries

1 tbsp honey

1 tbsp chia seeds (optional, for added texture and nutrients)

1 tsp lemon zest (optional, for extra flavor)

Instructions:

1. Spoon Greek yogurt into bowls.

2. Top with fresh blueberries.

3. Drizzle with honey.

4. Sprinkle chia seeds and lemon zest if using.

5. Serve immediately or refrigerate until ready to eat.

Nutritional Information (per serving):

Calories: 180 kcal

Protein: 10 g

Fat: 3 g

Carbohydrates: 30 g

Sodium: 70 mg

Explanation:

Greek yogurt is an excellent source of probiotics, which help restore beneficial bacteria in the gut, especially important after fasting. It is also rich in protein, making it a nutritious and filling option. Blueberries add natural sweetness and antioxidants, supporting overall health and aiding in digestion. Honey provides a touch of natural sweetness and has antibacterial properties, which can also aid digestion. Chia seeds add fiber and omega3 fatty acids, further enhancing the nutritional profile of the meal. This simple yet nutrientdense dish is ideal for reintroducing foods and supporting digestive health postfast.

MASHED SWEET POTATOES WITH BONE BROTH

Servings: 4

Prep Time: 10 minutes

Cook Time: 25 minutes

Ingredients:

4 medium sweet potatoes, peeled and cubed

1 cup bone broth (chicken or beef)

2 tbsp unsalted butter or ghee

1/4 cup milk (dairy or nondairy)

1/2 tsp ground cinnamon

Salt and pepper to taste

Chopped fresh parsley for garnish (optional)

Instructions:

1. Place sweet potato cubes in a large pot and cover with water. Bring to a boil and cook until tender, about 1520 minutes.

2. Drain the sweet potatoes and return them to the pot.

3. Add bone broth, butter or ghee, and milk. Mash the sweet potatoes with a potato masher or use an immersion blender for a smoother texture.

4. Stir in ground cinnamon, and season with salt and pepper to taste.

5. Garnish with fresh parsley if desired, and serve warm.

Nutritional Information (per serving):

Calories: 180 kcal

Protein: 4 g

Fat: 7 g

Carbohydrates: 26 g

Sodium: 200 mg

Explanation:

Sweet potatoes are rich in vitamins A and C, fiber, and antioxidants, making them a nourishing choice for gut healing. Bone broth, simmered from animal bones and connective tissue, is packed with collagen, gelatin, and amino acids, which can help repair and soothe the gut lining. The combination of these ingredients creates a comforting, nutrientdense dish that supports digestive health and recovery postfast. The addition of butter or ghee adds healthy fats that aid in the absorption of fatsoluble vitamins, while cinnamon provides antiinflammatory benefits. This recipe is designed to be easy on the digestive system while offering essential nutrients for overall wellness.

Roasted Carrot Puree with Ginger and Turmeric

Servings: 4

Prep Time: 15 minutes

Cook Time: 30 minutes

Ingredients:

6 large carrots, peeled and chopped

1 tbsp olive oil

1 tsp ground turmeric

1/2 tsp ground ginger

Salt and pepper to taste

1/4 cup vegetable broth or water

Fresh cilantro for garnish (optional)

Instructions:

1. Preheat the oven to 400°F (200°C).

2. Toss the chopped carrots with olive oil, turmeric, ginger, salt, and pepper. Spread them out in a single layer on a baking sheet.

3. Roast in the oven for 2530 minutes, or until the carrots are tender and lightly caramelized.

4. Transfer the roasted carrots to a blender or food processor. Add vegetable broth or water and blend until smooth.

5. Adjust seasoning as needed and garnish with fresh cilantro if desired. Serve warm.

Nutritional Information (per serving):

Calories: 130 kcal

Protein: 2 g

Fat: 5 g

Carbohydrates: 20 g

Sodium: 150 mg

Explanation:

Carrots are rich in betacarotene, fiber, and antioxidants, which support digestive health and immune function. Roasting carrots enhances their natural sweetness and can make them easier to digest. Ginger and turmeric are wellknown for their antiinflammatory and gutsoothing properties, helping to reduce inflammation and support digestion. Turmeric contains curcumin, a powerful antiinflammatory compound that can aid in gut healing. This dish is not only flavorful but also provides a soothing and restorative option for reintroducing solid foods after fasting. The smooth puree is gentle on the stomach and offers a rich source of nutrients to help restore balance and support recovery.

Light Protein Options

Poached Eggs with Sautéed Spinach

Servings: 2

Prep Time: 10 minutes

Cook Time: 10 minutes

Ingredients:

4 large eggs

2 cups fresh spinach, washed and trimmed

1 tbsp olive oil

1 clove garlic, minced

Salt and pepper to taste

Lemon juice (optional, for seasoning)

Instructions:

1. Bring a pot of water to a gentle simmer. Add a splash of vinegar if desired (to help the eggs hold their shape).

2. Crack each egg into a small bowl or cup. Gently slide each egg into the simmering water, one at a time.

3. Poach the eggs for 34 minutes, until the whites are set but the yolks are still runny. Remove with a slotted spoon and drain on a paper towel.

4. Meanwhile, heat olive oil in a skillet over medium heat. Add minced garlic and sauté until fragrant, about 1 minute.

5. Add spinach to the skillet and cook until wilted, about 23 minutes. Season with salt and pepper to taste.

6. Serve the poached eggs on a plate alongside the sautéed spinach. Optionally, drizzle with a bit of lemon juice for extra flavor.

Nutritional Information (per serving):

Calories: 280 kcal

Protein: 20 g

Fat: 18 g

Carbohydrates: 5 g

Sodium: 220 mg

Explanation:

Poached eggs are an excellent source of highquality protein and essential nutrients such as vitamins B12 and D, and choline, which supports brain health. Eggs are easy to digest, making them a suitable option for reintroducing protein into your diet postfast. Sautéed spinach adds a dose of iron, vitamins A and C, and fiber. Spinach is also rich in antioxidants, which can aid in reducing inflammation and supporting overall recovery. Olive oil provides healthy fats, which are important for cellular health and absorption of fatsoluble vitamins. This dish is designed to be gentle on the digestive system while providing necessary protein and nutrients to support healing after fasting.

GRILLED CHICKEN WITH STEAMED CAULIFLOWER

Servings: 2

Prep Time: 15 minutes

Cook Time: 20 minutes

Ingredients:

2 boneless, skinless chicken breasts

1 tbsp olive oil

1 tsp dried thyme

1/2 tsp garlic powder

Salt and pepper to taste

1 small head of cauliflower, cut into florets

1 tbsp lemon juice (optional)

Instructions:

1. Preheat the grill to mediumhigh heat.

2. Brush the chicken breasts with olive oil and season with dried thyme, garlic powder, salt, and pepper.

3. Grill the chicken for 67 minutes on each side, or until the internal temperature reaches 165°F (75°C) and the juices run clear.

4. While the chicken is grilling, steam the cauliflower florets. Place them in a steamer basket over boiling water and cook for 710 minutes, or until tender.

5. Once cooked, season the cauliflower with a bit of salt and pepper, and drizzle with lemon juice if desired.

6. Serve the grilled chicken alongside the steamed cauliflower.

Nutritional Information (per serving):

Calories: 300 kcal

Protein: 30 g

Fat: 15 g

Carbohydrates: 10 g

Sodium: 180 mg

Explanation:

Grilled chicken is a lean protein source that is easy to digest and helps rebuild muscle and tissue postfast. Chicken breast is low in fat and high in essential amino acids, which are crucial for recovery and repair. Cauliflower is a lowcalorie, nutrientdense vegetable that provides vitamins C and K, fiber, and antioxidants. Steaming cauliflower helps retain its nutrients while making it easy on the digestive system. Olive oil adds a touch of healthy fat, which supports overall cell function and aids in the absorption of fatsoluble vitamins. This meal is designed to be nourishing, balanced, and easy to digest, making it ideal for reintroducing protein and vegetables into your diet following a fasting period.

Chapter 9

LongTerm Maintenance Recipes

Balanced Breakfasts

Chia Pudding with Almond Milk and Berries

Servings: 2

Prep Time: 10 minutes

Cook Time: None (requires refrigeration)

Ingredients:

1/4 cup chia seeds

1 cup unsweetened almond milk

1 tbsp maple syrup or honey (optional)

1/2 tsp vanilla extract

1/2 cup mixed berries (such as strawberries, blueberries, and raspberries)

Instructions:

1. In a bowl, combine chia seeds, almond milk, maple syrup (if using), and vanilla extract. Stir well to ensure the chia seeds are evenly distributed.

2. Cover the bowl and refrigerate for at least 4 hours, or overnight. Stir occasionally if possible to prevent the chia seeds from clumping.

3. Once the pudding has thickened and the chia seeds have absorbed the liquid, divide it into two serving bowls.

4. Top with mixed berries before serving.

Nutritional Information (per serving):

Calories: 250 kcal

Protein: 7 g

Fat: 12 g

Carbohydrates: 30 g

Fiber: 11 g

Sodium: 100 mg

Explanation:

Chia pudding is an excellent breakfast option for longterm maintenance as it provides a balanced mix of protein, healthy fats, and fiber. Chia seeds are a great source of omega3 fatty acids, which are important for heart health, and they also help to keep you full longer due to their high fiber content. Almond milk keeps the dish light and low in calories while adding a subtle nutty flavor. Berries provide antioxidants and additional fiber, helping to support overall health and digestion. This breakfast is easy to prepare and perfect for a quick, nutritious start to the day.

OVERNIGHT OATS WITH BANANA AND CHIA SEEDS

Servings: 2

Prep Time: 5 minutes

Cook Time: None (requires refrigeration)

Ingredients:

1/2 cup rolled oats

1/2 cup milk (dairy or nondairy)

1/4 cup Greek yogurt

1 tbsp chia seeds

1 ripe banana, sliced

1 tbsp honey or maple syrup (optional)

1/2 tsp cinnamon

Instructions:

1. In a jar or bowl, combine rolled oats, milk, Greek yogurt, chia seeds, and honey or maple syrup (if using). Mix well.

2. Stir in the cinnamon.

3. Cover and refrigerate overnight, or for at least 4 hours.

4. In the morning, stir the oats and top with sliced banana before serving.

Nutritional Information (per serving):

Calories: 280 kcal

Protein: 10 g

Fat: 7 g

Carbohydrates: 45 g

Fiber: 6 g

Sodium: 120 mg

Explanation:

Overnight oats are a convenient and nutritious breakfast choice that can support longterm maintenance by offering a good mix of protein, carbohydrates, and fiber. Rolled oats are a whole grain that provides sustained energy, while Greek yogurt adds protein and probiotics for digestive health. Chia seeds enhance the fiber content and contribute omega3 fatty acids. The banana adds natural sweetness and potassium, which helps maintain electrolyte balance. This dish is easy to prepare in advance, making it a practical option for busy mornings.

Grilled Chicken Salad with Olive Oil and Lemon

Servings: 2

Prep Time: 15 minutes

Cook Time: 10 minutes

Ingredients:

2 boneless, skinless chicken breasts

1 tbsp olive oil

Juice of 1 lemon

1 tsp dried oregano

Salt and pepper to taste

4 cups mixed salad greens (such as arugula, spinach, and romaine)

1/2 cup cherry tomatoes, halved

1/4 cup red onion, thinly sliced

1/4 cup cucumber, sliced

1/4 cup feta cheese, crumbled (optional)

Instructions:

1. Preheat grill or grill pan over medium heat.

2. Brush chicken breasts with olive oil, lemon juice, oregano, salt, and pepper.

3. Grill chicken for about 5 minutes per side or until the internal temperature reaches 165°F (74°C) and juices run clear.

4. Remove chicken from the grill and let it rest for 5 minutes before slicing.

5. While chicken rests, assemble the salad: Arrange the mixed greens, cherry tomatoes, red onion, and cucumber on plates.

6. Slice the grilled chicken and place it on top of the salad.

7. Sprinkle with feta cheese, if desired, and drizzle with additional olive oil and lemon juice if preferred.

Nutritional Information (per serving):

Calories: 350 kcal

Protein: 35 g

Fat: 18 g

Carbohydrates: 12 g

Fiber: 4 g

Sodium: 500 mg

Explanation:

This Grilled Chicken Salad is an ideal choice for maintaining health due to its wellbalanced combination of lean protein, healthy fats, and fresh vegetables. Chicken breast is a highquality protein source that supports muscle maintenance and repair, while olive oil provides monounsaturated fats that promote heart health. Lemon juice adds a refreshing tang while also contributing vitamin C, which is essential for immune function. The mixed greens and vegetables in the salad offer vitamins, minerals, and fiber, which are crucial for overall health and digestive function. This meal is light yet filling, making it a great option for a satisfying lunch that supports longterm wellness.

BLACK BEAN AND QUINOA BOWL WITH AVOCADO

Servings: 2

Prep Time: 15 minutes

Cook Time: 20 minutes

Ingredients:

1 cup cooked quinoa

1 can (15 oz) black beans, drained and rinsed

1 cup corn kernels (fresh or frozen)

1 red bell pepper, diced

1 avocado, sliced

1/4 cup cilantro, chopped

Juice of 1 lime

1 tbsp olive oil

Salt and pepper to taste

Instructions:

1. In a large bowl, combine cooked quinoa, black beans, corn, and diced red bell pepper.

2. In a small bowl, whisk together lime juice, olive oil, salt, and pepper.

3. Pour the lime dressing over the quinoa mixture and toss to combine.

4. Divide the quinoa and bean mixture into two bowls.

5. Top each bowl with sliced avocado and chopped cilantro.

Nutritional Information (per serving):

Calories: 400 kcal

Protein: 15 g

Fat: 15 g

Carbohydrates: 55 g

Fiber: 12 g

Sodium: 200 mg

Explanation:

The Black Bean and Quinoa Bowl is a nutrientdense lunch option that combines plantbased protein with complex carbohydrates and healthy fats. Quinoa and black beans provide a complete protein source, essential for maintaining muscle mass and overall health. Black beans are also rich in fiber, which aids digestion and helps regulate blood sugar levels. Corn and red bell peppers add a touch of sweetness and a boost of vitamins, while avocado contributes healthy monounsaturated fats and additional fiber. Cilantro and lime juice enhance the flavor while offering antioxidants and vitamin C. This dish is both satisfying and nutritious, making it an excellent choice for longterm health maintenance.

Baked Salmon with Sweet Potato and Asparagus

Servings: 2

Prep Time: 15 minutes

Cook Time: 25 minutes

Ingredients:

2 salmon fillets (6 oz each)

1 large sweet potato, peeled and cut into cubes

1 bunch asparagus, trimmed

2 tbsp olive oil

1 tsp dried thyme

1 tsp paprika

2 cloves garlic, minced

Salt and pepper to taste

Lemon wedges for serving

Instructions:

1. Preheat the oven to 400°F (200°C).

2. Toss sweet potato cubes with 1 tbsp olive oil, thyme, paprika, salt, and pepper. Spread on a baking sheet.

3. Bake sweet potatoes in the preheated oven for 15 minutes.

4. While sweet potatoes are baking, toss asparagus with remaining olive oil, garlic, salt, and pepper.

5. After 15 minutes, remove the baking sheet, and add the asparagus to the sheet with sweet potatoes.

6. Place salmon fillets on top of the vegetables and season with additional salt and pepper.

7. Return to the oven and bake for an additional 1012 minutes, or until the salmon is cooked through and flakes easily with a fork.

8. Serve with lemon wedges on the side.

Nutritional Information (per serving):

Calories: 450 kcal

Protein: 35 g

Fat: 22 g

Carbohydrates: 35 g

Fiber: 6 g

Sodium: 150 mg

Explanation:

Baked Salmon with Sweet Potato and Asparagus is an excellent choice for a balanced dinner that supports longterm health. Salmon is rich in omega3 fatty acids, which are known for their antiinflammatory properties and benefits to heart health. It also provides highquality protein, essential for muscle maintenance and overall body repair. Sweet potatoes are a great source of complex carbohydrates and betacarotene, contributing to sustained energy levels and improved immune function. Asparagus adds additional fiber, vitamins, and antioxidants. This dish is baked with minimal added fat, utilizing olive oil for healthy fats and flavor. The combination of these ingredients not only makes for a delicious and satisfying meal but also provides a range of nutrients that support overall wellness and balance.

Tofu StirFry with Brown Rice and Vegetables

Servings: 2

Prep Time: 15 minutes

Cook Time: 20 minutes

Ingredients:

1 block firm tofu, drained and cubed

1 cup brown rice, cooked

1 red bell pepper, sliced

1 cup broccoli florets

1 cup snap peas

2 tbsp soy sauce (or tamari for glutenfree)

1 tbsp sesame oil

2 tbsp hoisin sauce

1 tbsp grated ginger

2 cloves garlic, minced

2 green onions, sliced

Sesame seeds for garnish (optional)

Instructions:

1. Heat sesame oil in a large skillet or wok over mediumhigh heat.

2. Add cubed tofu and cook until golden brown and crispy on all sides, about 710 minutes. Remove tofu from the skillet and set aside.

3. In the same skillet, add garlic and ginger, and sauté for 1 minute until fragrant.

4. Add red bell pepper, broccoli, and snap peas, and stirfry for 57 minutes until vegetables are tendercrisp.

5. Return tofu to the skillet and pour in soy sauce and hoisin sauce. Toss to coat the tofu and vegetables evenly.

6. Cook for an additional 2 minutes, allowing the sauce to slightly thicken.

7. Serve over cooked brown rice and garnish with sliced green onions and sesame seeds if desired.

Nutritional Information (per serving):

Calories: 400 kcal

Protein: 20 g

Fat: 15 g

Carbohydrates: 45 g

Fiber: 8 g

Sodium: 600 mg

Explanation:

Tofu StirFry with Brown Rice and Vegetables is a nutrientrich meal that provides a balanced mix of protein, carbohydrates, and fats. Tofu is an excellent plantbased protein source that supports muscle repair and growth, while brown rice offers whole grains that contribute to sustained energy and digestive health. The variety of vegetables—red bell pepper, broccoli, and snap peas—adds essential vitamins, minerals, and antioxidants that help protect against chronic diseases and support overall health.

Stirfrying with sesame oil and a touch of soy sauce and hoisin sauce enhances the flavor while keeping the dish light and nutritious. This meal is a perfect option for maintaining longterm health, offering a satisfying and wholesome dinner that aligns with dietary goals and supports overall wellbeing.

Chapter 10

Snack Ideas for Refeeding

RICE CAKES WITH AVOCADO

Servings: 1

Prep Time: 5 minutes

Cook Time: 0 minutes

Ingredients:

2 plain rice cakes

1 ripe avocado

1 tbsp lemon juice

Salt and pepper to taste

Red pepper flakes or chopped fresh herbs for garnish (optional)

Instructions:

1. In a bowl, mash the avocado with a fork until smooth.

2. Stir in lemon juice, salt, and pepper to taste.

3. Spread the mashed avocado evenly over the rice cakes.

4. Garnish with red pepper flakes or fresh herbs if desired.

Nutritional Information (per serving):

Calories: 250 kcal

Protein: 4 g

Fat: 18 g

Carbohydrates: 22 g

Fiber: 8 g

Sodium: 10 mg

Explanation:

Rice Cakes with Avocado is a simple yet nutritious snack perfect for refeeding. Rice cakes are a lowcalorie, easily digestible base that provides carbohydrates for energy. The avocado topping adds healthy fats and a creamy texture while supplying essential nutrients like potassium, fiber, and monounsaturated fats. The lemon juice enhances flavor and adds a fresh, zesty touch. This snack is both satisfying and easy on the digestive system, making it an excellent choice for reintroducing solid foods after a fast.

CUCUMBER SLICES WITH GREEK YOGURT

Servings: 1

Prep Time: 5 minutes

Cook Time: 0 minutes

Ingredients:

1 cucumber, sliced into rounds

1/2 cup Greek yogurt (plain)

1 tbsp fresh dill, chopped (or mint for a different flavor)

1 tbsp lemon juice

Salt and pepper to taste

Instructions:

1. Arrange cucumber slices on a plate.

2. In a small bowl, mix Greek yogurt with dill, lemon juice, salt, and pepper.

3. Serve the yogurt mixture as a dip alongside the cucumber slices.

Nutritional Information (per serving):

Calories: 120 kcal

Protein: 8 g

Fat: 3 g

Carbohydrates: 15 g

Fiber: 2 g

Sodium: 50 mg

Explanation:

Cucumber Slices with Greek Yogurt is a refreshing and light snack ideal for refeeding. Cucumbers are hydrating and low in calories, while Greek yogurt provides protein and probiotics beneficial for gut health. The addition of fresh dill or mint and a splash of lemon juice enhances the flavor profile without adding excessive calories. This snack supports a gentle transition back to solid foods, providing essential nutrients and aiding in digestion with a cool, crisp texture.

Apple Slices with Almond Butter

Servings: 1

Prep Time: 5 minutes

Cook Time: 0 minutes

Ingredients:

1 medium apple

2 tbsp almond butter

1/2 tsp cinnamon (optional)

1 tsp honey or maple syrup (optional)

Instructions:

1. Core and slice the apple into thin wedges.

2. Arrange apple slices on a plate.

3. Serve with almond butter for dipping.

4. Sprinkle with cinnamon or drizzle with honey/maple syrup if desired.

Nutritional Information (per serving):

Calories: 210 kcal

Protein: 4 g

Fat: 14 g

Carbohydrates: 24 g

Fiber: 5 g

Sodium: 0 mg

Explanation:

Apple Slices with Almond Butter is a nutritious and satisfying snack ideal for refeeding after a fast. Apples provide natural sweetness, fiber, and essential vitamins, while almond butter adds healthy fats, protein, and a creamy texture. The combination of apple and almond butter offers a balance of macronutrients that supports energy levels and helps stabilize blood sugar. The optional cinnamon and honey or maple syrup enhance the flavor profile, adding a touch of sweetness and a hint of spice. This snack is both easy to prepare and gentle on the digestive system, making it a great option for gradually reintroducing foods.

BANANA AND NUT BUTTER

Servings: 1

Prep Time: 5 minutes

Cook Time: 0 minutes

Ingredients:

1 ripe banana

2 tbsp nut butter (e.g., almond, cashew, or peanut)

1/2 tbsp chia seeds (optional)

A sprinkle of sea salt (optional)

Instructions:

1. Peel and slice the banana into thin rounds.

2. Spread nut butter evenly over banana slices or dip each slice into the nut butter.

3. Sprinkle with chia seeds and a pinch of sea salt if desired.

Nutritional Information (per serving):

Calories: 220 kcal

Protein: 5 g

Fat: 12 g

Carbohydrates: 26 g

Fiber: 5 g

Sodium: 70 mg

Explanation:

Banana and Nut Butter is a quick, nutrientrich snack that provides a good balance of carbohydrates, protein, and healthy fats. Bananas are rich in potassium, which helps regulate fluid balance and muscle function, while nut butter adds protein and healthy fats to keep you satisfied. Chia seeds, if added, provide additional fiber, omega3 fatty acids, and a pleasant crunch. This snack is ideal for refeeding, offering both energy and essential nutrients while being easy to digest and enjoyable.

STEAMED EDAMAME WITH SEA SALT

Servings: 1

Prep Time: 5 minutes

Cook Time: 5 minutes

Ingredients:

1 cup shelled edamame (fresh or frozen)

1/2 tsp sea salt

1/2 tsp olive oil (optional)

Instructions:

1. Steam edamame in a steamer basket over boiling water for 5 minutes, or until tender.

2. Remove from heat and sprinkle with sea salt. Toss with olive oil if desired.

Nutritional Information (per serving):

Calories: 130 kcal

Protein: 12 g

Fat: 5 g

Carbohydrates: 12 g

Fiber: 6 g

Sodium: 200 mg

Explanation:

Steamed Edamame with Sea Salt is a proteinpacked snack that is both satisfying and easy on the digestive system. Edamame, young soybeans, provide a rich source of plantbased protein, fiber, and essential vitamins and minerals. The steaming process helps retain the beans' nutrients while making them soft and easy to digest. A light sprinkle of sea salt enhances the flavor without overwhelming the taste. This snack is an excellent choice for those reintroducing foods postfast, as it offers a nutrientdense, lowcalorie option that supports muscle repair and overall recovery.

SOFTBOILED EGG WITH SPINACH

Servings: 1

Prep Time: 5 minutes

Cook Time: 10 minutes

Ingredients:

1 large egg

1 cup fresh spinach leaves

1/2 tsp olive oil (optional)

Salt and pepper to taste

Instructions:

1. Bring a small pot of water to a boil.

2. Gently add the egg and boil for 9 minutes.

3. Transfer the egg to a bowl of ice water and let it cool for a few minutes. Peel the egg.

4. In a pan, heat olive oil over medium heat and sauté spinach until wilted, about 2 minutes.

5. Season spinach with salt and pepper, and serve alongside the peeled softboiled egg.

Nutritional Information (per serving):

Calories: 150 kcal

Protein: 12 g

Fat: 10 g

Carbohydrates: 2 g

Fiber: 1 g

Sodium: 200 mg

Explanation:

SoftBoiled Egg with Spinach is a nutrientdense snack ideal for refeeding. The softboiled egg provides highquality protein, healthy fats, and essential vitamins such as B12 and choline. Spinach is rich in iron, vitamins A and C, and antioxidants that support overall health. This dish is easy to prepare, easy to digest, and offers a balanced combination of protein and vegetables, making it a great choice for gradually reintroducing food after a fast.

HUMMUS WITH CARROT STICKS

Servings: 1

Prep Time: 5 minutes

Cook Time: 0 minutes

Ingredients:

1/2 cup hummus (storebought or homemade)

1 medium carrot, peeled and cut into sticks

Instructions:

1. Arrange carrot sticks on a plate.

2. Serve with hummus for dipping.

Nutritional Information (per serving):

Calories: 180 kcal

Protein: 6 g

Fat: 10 g

Carbohydrates: 20 g

Fiber: 5 g

Sodium: 280 mg

Explanation:

Hummus with Carrot Sticks is a simple yet nourishing snack that combines the fiber and vitamins of carrots with the protein and healthy fats of hummus. Carrots are an excellent source of betacarotene, which supports eye health, while hummus provides protein and healthy fats from chickpeas and olive oil. This snack is easy to digest, low in calories, and provides a satisfying crunch, making it ideal for refeeding.

Cottage Cheese with Pineapple

Servings: 1

Prep Time: 5 minutes

Cook Time: 0 minutes

Ingredients:

1/2 cup lowfat cottage cheese

1/4 cup pineapple chunks (fresh or canned in juice, drained)

Instructions:

1. Combine cottage cheese and pineapple chunks in a bowl.

2. Stir gently and serve.

Nutritional Information (per serving):

Calories: 150 kcal

Protein: 14 g

Fat: 2 g

Carbohydrates: 20 g

Fiber: 1 g

Sodium: 300 mg

Explanation:

Cottage Cheese with Pineapple is a refreshing and proteinrich snack suitable for postfasting. Cottage cheese is high in protein and calcium, supporting muscle repair and bone health, while pineapple adds natural sweetness, vitamin C, and digestive enzymes that can aid in digestion. This combination provides a balanced mix of protein and carbohydrates, making it a nourishing option for those reintroducing foods after a fast.

ALMONDS AND DRIED FRUIT MIX

Servings: 1

Prep Time: 5 minutes

Cook Time: 0 minutes

Ingredients:

1/4 cup raw almonds

1/4 cup dried fruit (such as raisins, cranberries, or apricots)

Instructions:

1. Combine almonds and dried fruit in a bowl.

2. Mix well and serve.

Nutritional Information (per serving):

Calories: 210 kcal

Protein: 5 g

Fat: 12 g

Carbohydrates: 23 g

Fiber: 4 g

Sodium: 0 mg

Explanation:

Almonds and Dried Fruit Mix is a convenient and nutrientdense snack ideal for postfasting refeeding. Almonds provide healthy fats, protein, and vitamin E, which are crucial for cellular repair and energy. They also contribute magnesium and fiber, which support digestive health. Dried fruit adds natural sweetness and essential vitamins and minerals, such as iron and potassium, while offering a quick source of energy. This mix is both satisfying and easy to digest, making it a balanced choice for reintroducing solid foods. However, it should be consumed in moderation due to the high calorie and sugar content from the dried fruit.

Baked Apple with Cinnamon

Servings: 1

Prep Time: 10 minutes

Cook Time: 20 minutes

Ingredients:

1 medium apple, cored and sliced

1/2 tsp ground cinnamon

1/2 tsp honey or maple syrup (optional)

Instructions:

1. Preheat the oven to 350°F (175°C).

2. Arrange apple slices on a baking sheet or in a baking dish.

3. Sprinkle with ground cinnamon. Drizzle with honey or maple syrup if desired.

4. Bake for 20 minutes, or until apples are tender and lightly caramelized.

5. Serve warm.

Nutritional Information (per serving):

Calories: 120 kcal

Protein: 0 g

Fat: 0 g

Carbohydrates: 31 g

Fiber: 5 g

Sodium: 0 mg

Explanation:

Baked Apple with Cinnamon is a comforting and easily digestible snack perfect for postfasting. Apples are a good source of dietary fiber, which helps with digestion and provides sustained energy. Cinnamon adds a flavorful touch and has antioxidant properties that can aid in metabolism and blood sugar regulation. Baking apples enhances their natural sweetness while making them tender and easy to digest. This snack is low in fat and protein, making it a gentle choice for reintroducing food while providing essential nutrients and a pleasant taste experience.

Chapter 11

Hydrating Herbal Teas and Drinks (10 Recipes)

GINGER AND LEMON TEA

Servings: 1

Prep Time: 5 minutes

Cook Time: 10 minutes

Ingredients:

1 inch fresh ginger root, peeled and sliced

1 lemon, juiced

1 tsp honey (optional)

2 cups water

Instructions:

1. Boil water in a small saucepan.

2. Add ginger slices and let simmer for 5–10 minutes.

3. Remove from heat and strain the ginger pieces.

4. Stir in fresh lemon juice and honey if desired.

5. Serve warm.

Explanation:

Ginger and lemon tea is a hydrating, antiinflammatory drink that aids in digestion and boosts the immune system. Ginger helps to soothe the stomach, while lemon adds a refreshing taste and a dose of vitamin C. It's perfect for postfasting as it helps gently reintroduce flavors and supports detoxification.

Peppermint Tea with Honey

Servings: 1

Prep Time: 5 minutes

Cook Time: 5 minutes

Ingredients:

1 peppermint tea bag or 1 tbsp dried peppermint leaves

1 tsp honey (optional)

1 cup boiling water

Instructions:

1. Steep the peppermint tea bag or leaves in boiling water for 5 minutes.

2. Remove the tea bag or strain the leaves.

3. Stir in honey if desired.

4. Serve warm.

Explanation:

Peppermint tea is known for its soothing effects on digestion and its ability to alleviate bloating and discomfort. It's caffeinefree, making it a gentle, calming drink for pre and postfast hydration. Honey adds a mild sweetness and antibacterial properties, but it can be omitted for a pure, clean flavor.

Chamomile Tea with Lavender

Servings: 1

Prep Time: 5 minutes

Cook Time: 5 minutes

Ingredients:

1 chamomile tea bag or 1 tbsp dried chamomile flowers

1 tsp dried lavender

1 cup boiling water

Instructions:

1. Steep the chamomile and lavender in boiling water for 5 minutes.

2. Strain the herbs or remove the tea bag.

3. Serve warm.

Explanation:

Chamomile tea with lavender is a relaxing blend that promotes restfulness and reduces anxiety, making it an ideal choice during or after a water fast. Chamomile is known for its calming properties, while lavender adds a floral aroma and enhances relaxation. This combination helps soothe the mind and body, aiding in stress relief during the fasting process.

Warm Lemon Water with Honey

Servings: 1

Prep Time: 5 minutes

Cook Time: 0 minutes

Ingredients:

1 cup warm water (not boiling)

1 tbsp fresh lemon juice (about 1/2 lemon)

1 tsp raw honey (optional)

Instructions:

1. Warm water until it's just comfortably hot but not boiling.

2. Add the fresh lemon juice to the water and stir.

3. Mix in honey if you prefer a sweetener.

4. Sip slowly, ideally first thing in the morning on an empty stomach.

Explanation:

Warm lemon water with honey is a simple but powerful drink that promotes hydration, supports digestion, and provides a gentle detox. Lemon is packed with vitamin C, which helps boost the immune system and supports skin health. The acidity of lemon also helps to stimulate bile production, aiding in digestion and detoxification, which is especially beneficial after fasting.

Honey, if used, offers antibacterial and antiviral properties, providing a natural boost to immune defenses. It also soothes the digestive system and may help alleviate acid reflux by balancing pH levels in the stomach. Drinking warm lemon water upon waking hydrates the body after hours of fasting (during sleep) and prepares the digestive system for the day. It also alkalizes the body, balancing out the acidity of a modern diet, while the warmth of the drink aids digestion.

This drink is an excellent option for reintroducing your digestive system to food after fasting, as it is light, soothing, and hydrating.

Green Tea with Mint

Servings: 1

Prep Time: 5 minutes

Cook Time: 5 minutes

Ingredients:

1 green tea bag or 1 tsp loose green tea

A few fresh mint leaves

1 cup hot water

Honey (optional)

Instructions:

1. Boil water and let it cool slightly before pouring it over the green tea bag or loose leaves (green tea can turn bitter if brewed in boiling water).

2. Add mint leaves while the tea steeps for 35 minutes.

3. Remove the tea bag or strain the leaves.

4. Sweeten with honey if desired, and enjoy.

Explanation:

Green tea with mint is a refreshing and light drink that combines the antioxidant properties of green tea with the soothing and digestiveenhancing benefits of mint. Green tea contains catechins, which are powerful antioxidants that support overall health, boost metabolism, and improve brain function. Its moderate caffeine content provides a gentle energy lift without the crash of coffee, making it ideal for postfast recovery.

Mint is known for its ability to soothe digestive discomfort, reduce nausea, and promote digestion. Adding mint to green tea creates a calming, refreshing drink that helps hydrate the body, improves gut health, and provides mental clarity. This tea is an excellent choice for transitioning back into a regular eating routine after fasting, as it is gentle on the stomach and supports the digestive process.

HIBISCUS ICED TEA

Servings: 2

Prep Time: 10 minutes

Cook Time: 5 minutes

Ingredients:

2 tbsp dried hibiscus flowers or 2 hibiscus tea bags

4 cups water

1 tbsp honey or agave syrup (optional)

Ice cubes

Fresh mint leaves (optional, for garnish)

Instructions:

1. Bring 4 cups of water to a boil, then add hibiscus flowers or tea bags.

2. Let it steep for 510 minutes depending on your desired strength.

3. Strain the tea or remove the tea bags, and let the tea cool.

4. Add honey or sweetener if desired.

5. Pour the tea over ice and garnish with fresh mint leaves if using.

Explanation:

Hibiscus iced tea is not only a vibrant, tangy, and refreshing drink, but it's also packed with health benefits, particularly for postfast hydration. Hibiscus tea is known for its high antioxidant content, which helps combat oxidative stress and inflammation in the body. It's also rich in vitamin C, supporting immune function and skin health.

A key benefit of hibiscus tea is its ability to help lower blood pressure, making it a hearthealthy option. Its naturally tart flavor can satisfy the palate without the need for added sugar, though a touch of honey or agave can balance the flavor if needed. The cooling, refreshing nature of hibiscus tea makes it a perfect hydrating option after fasting, especially during warm weather, as it replenishes lost fluids and vital nutrients without adding excess calories.

TURMERIC GOLDEN MILK

Servings: 1

Prep Time: 5 minutes

Cook Time: 5 minutes

Ingredients:

1 cup unsweetened almond milk (or any plantbased milk)

1/2 tsp ground turmeric

1/4 tsp ground ginger or 1/2 inch fresh ginger root, sliced

A pinch of black pepper (to enhance turmeric absorption)

1 tsp honey or maple syrup (optional)

A pinch of cinnamon (optional)

Instructions:

1. Heat the almond milk in a small saucepan over medium heat.

2. Add turmeric, ginger, black pepper, and cinnamon, stirring to combine.

3. Simmer for 5 minutes, stirring occasionally.

4. Remove from heat and strain if using fresh ginger.

5. Stir in honey or maple syrup to taste, if desired.

6. Serve warm.

Explanation:

Turmeric golden milk, also known as "golden latte," is a soothing and nutrientrich drink that harnesses the antiinflammatory power of turmeric. Turmeric contains curcumin, a compound that is wellknown for its ability to reduce inflammation, improve brain function, and support heart health. However, curcumin is poorly absorbed on its own, which is why black pepper is added to enhance its bioavailability.

Ginger complements turmeric's antiinflammatory properties and adds a warming, digestiveaid quality to the drink. Almond milk (or another plantbased milk) provides a creamy base that is easy on the stomach and offers essential nutrients like vitamin E and calcium. Cinnamon, if added, adds a touch of warmth and natural sweetness while also helping to regulate blood sugar levels.

Golden milk is particularly restorative after fasting because of its ability to soothe the digestive system, reduce inflammation, and support recovery. It also helps relax the body, making it an excellent choice to enjoy in the evening or before bedtime. It's a nourishing and comforting drink that promotes overall wellness and healing, especially after periods of fasting or dietary restriction.

WARM CINNAMON WATER

Servings: 1

Prep Time: 2 minutes

Cook Time: 5 minutes

Ingredients:

1 cinnamon stick (or 1/2 tsp ground cinnamon)

1 cup water

Honey or lemon (optional)

Instructions:

1. Boil the water in a small saucepan.

2. Add the cinnamon stick (or ground cinnamon) to the water and let it simmer for 5 minutes.

3. Remove the cinnamon stick or let the ground cinnamon settle at the bottom.

4. Stir in honey or lemon for taste, if desired.

5. Sip slowly and enjoy the warming effects.

Explanation:

Warm cinnamon water is a comforting and healthboosting beverage known for its digestive and metabolic benefits. Cinnamon has been used in traditional medicine for centuries due to its powerful antioxidant and antiinflammatory properties. It is particularly effective in regulating blood sugar levels, making it a great drink for those coming off a fast when blood sugar may need stabilization.

Drinking cinnamon water can help reduce cravings and improve insulin sensitivity, which is especially useful in maintaining longterm health after fasting. Cinnamon also stimulates circulation and digestion, helping the body to recover from the fasting process more efficiently. Adding a touch of honey provides additional soothing properties and supports immune health, while lemon adds a burst of vitamin C, aiding in digestion and detoxification.

Rooibos Tea with Vanilla

Servings: 1

Prep Time: 3 minutes

Cook Time: 5 minutes

Ingredients:

1 rooibos tea bag (or 1 tsp loose rooibos tea)

1 cup boiling water

1/4 tsp vanilla extract (or a vanilla pod)

Honey or agave syrup (optional)

Instructions:

1. Steep the rooibos tea in boiling water for 5 minutes.

2. Stir in the vanilla extract or steep a vanilla pod with the tea for a more natural flavor.

3. Sweeten with honey or agave syrup if desired.

4. Enjoy hot or over ice for a refreshing alternative.

Explanation:

Rooibos tea, a naturally caffeinefree herbal tea from South Africa, is known for its high levels of antioxidants, including aspalathin and quercetin, which help reduce oxidative stress in the body. It also contains minerals like calcium, magnesium, and potassium, which are important for rebalancing the body's electrolytes after a fast. Rooibos is gentle on the digestive system, making it an excellent postfast drink.

Adding vanilla enhances the soothing properties of rooibos, offering a rich, aromatic flavor that promotes relaxation. Vanilla has antioxidant properties as well and is known to reduce inflammation and improve mood. This tea is ideal for sipping in the evening when you want a calming, hydrating drink that supports the body's natural recovery processes without the stimulant effects of caffeine.

FENNEL SEED INFUSION

Servings: 1

Prep Time: 2 minutes

Cook Time: 5 minutes

Ingredients:

1 tsp fennel seeds

1 cup boiling water

Honey or lemon (optional)

Instructions:

1. Boil water and pour it over fennel seeds in a cup or teapot.

2. Let the seeds steep for 5 minutes, allowing their natural oils to release.

3. Strain the liquid into a cup.

4. Add honey or lemon for extra flavor, if desired.

5. Sip slowly, particularly after meals.

Explanation:

Fennel seed infusion is an ageold remedy for digestive issues, particularly bloating, gas, and indigestion. Fennel seeds contain volatile oils that relax the muscles in the digestive tract, making this drink an excellent choice for easing digestive discomfort after a fast. The infusion also helps stimulate digestion and detoxification, helping to flush out toxins that may have accumulated during fasting.

Fennel is rich in fiber, potassium, and magnesium, which support the body's recovery after fasting. It also has mild diuretic properties, helping reduce water retention and promoting gentle detoxification. This herbal infusion is calming and rejuvenating, making it a great addition to your refeeding period when the digestive system needs to adjust to solid foods again.

Chapter 11

Conclusion

Maintaining Health After Fasting

Integrating Balanced Eating Habits

Maintaining health after fasting requires a thoughtful approach to nutrition, hydration, and lifestyle habits. After a water fast, your body has gone through a period of rest and detoxification, and it is crucial to reintroduce foods gradually and with balance. The goal is to adopt sustainable eating habits that continue to support your health and prevent the negative effects of overeating or nutrient deficiencies.

Balanced eating habits include the incorporation of all essential macronutrients—proteins, fats, and carbohydrates—in proportions that suit your individual needs. After fasting, prioritize whole, unprocessed foods that provide vital nutrients. Include a variety of fruits, vegetables, lean proteins, healthy fats, and whole grains. These foods supply essential vitamins, minerals, and fiber that your body needs to maintain energy levels and overall health.

Key steps to integrating balanced eating habits:

1. Start with Light, Easily Digestible Foods: After fasting, your digestive system is sensitive, and it's important to ease into eating with simple foods. Begin with nutrientrich soups, broths, and soft fruits or vegetables. Avoid heavy meals that can overwhelm your stomach.

2. Focus on Nutrient Density: Rather than focusing solely on caloric intake, pay attention to the nutritional value of your food. Aim for meals rich in vitamins, minerals, antioxidants, and phytonutrients that nourish the body on a cellular level.

3. Stay Hydrated: Continue to drink plenty of water and consider incorporating hydrating teas or electrolyterich drinks to maintain balance. Proper hydration aids digestion and helps the body absorb nutrients more efficiently.

4. Avoid Processed and Sugary Foods: These can cause blood sugar spikes and lead to cravings or overeating. Stick to whole foods that nourish your body and provide longlasting energy.

5. Practice Portion Control: Eating smaller, balanced meals throughout the day helps prevent overloading your digestive system. Mindful eating habits can help prevent overeating and support healthy digestion.

How to Transition from Fasting to a Healthy Lifestyle

The transition from fasting back to regular eating and a healthy lifestyle is an essential step in reaping the longterm benefits of water fasting. While fasting helps reset your body, it's what you do after the fast that determines the lasting effects on your health. This transition period allows your body to adjust back to solid foods while maintaining the detox and healing processes that began during fasting.

1. Start Slow:

After fasting, your digestive system needs time to adjust. Start with small, light meals, such as soft vegetables, soups, and broths. Gradually introduce more solid foods over the course of several days. This approach allows your gut microbiome to rebuild and thrive without overburdening your digestive system.

2. Incorporate Regular Meals:

Once you've reintroduced solid foods, focus on maintaining a consistent meal schedule with balanced, nutritious meals. Incorporating three wellbalanced meals a day or smaller, more frequent meals ensures that your body is getting a steady supply of nutrients, avoiding the temptation to overeat or binge on unhealthy snacks.

3. Prioritize Gut Health:

To fully recover from fasting, pay attention to your gut health by including probiotic and prebiotic foods, such as yogurt, sauerkraut, and fiberrich vegetables. These foods help rebuild the beneficial bacteria in your digestive system, which supports overall health, immunity, and digestion.

4. Build Sustainable Habits:

Use fasting as a catalyst for adopting healthy habits. Instead of viewing fasting as a shortterm solution, integrate healthy habits into your everyday routine. This could mean adopting intermittent fasting, where you continue to have shorter periods of fasting (like 12 to 16 hours overnight) to maintain metabolic health.

5. Exercise Moderately:

After fasting, it's important to get back to physical activity, but start with gentle exercises like walking, yoga, or stretching. As your body gets stronger, incorporate more vigorous workouts such as strength training or cardio. Exercise not only helps maintain a healthy weight but also improves mood and overall wellbeing.

6. Mindful Eating:

Fasting can heighten your awareness of hunger and fullness signals. Use this awareness to practice mindful eating, where you pay attention to your body's cues and eat when truly hungry, not out of habit or emotional triggers. Chew slowly and savor your food, ensuring proper digestion and greater satisfaction from meals.

7. Avoid Unhealthy Habits:

Finally, steer clear of returning to unhealthy habits such as latenight snacking, consuming processed foods, or overeating. Stick to your new healthy routine, making the postfast lifestyle part of your longterm wellness plan.

The key to maintaining health after a water fast lies in a balanced and gradual approach to refeeding, followed by a sustainable longterm healthy lifestyle. By focusing on nutrientdense foods, proper hydration, regular exercise, and mindful eating, you can not only recover from fasting but also enjoy enhanced health and wellbeing. This transition period is crucial, and how you handle it sets the foundation for lasting results—whether it's better digestion, improved mental clarity, or stable energy levels.

Making Water Fasting Part of Your Wellness Journey

Water fasting can become an essential part of a holistic wellness journey when approached thoughtfully and with mindfulness. Integrating water fasting periodically into your routine can help reset your body, promote cellular repair, and enhance overall health. However, it's crucial to recognize that water fasting is not a onetime event or a quickfix solution, but rather a tool that complements a balanced, healthy lifestyle.

1. Establishing a Fasting Routine: One of the keys to making water fasting part of your wellness journey is to develop a consistent routine that works for your body. Many people find that fasting for 24 to 48 hours periodically—such as once a month or every few months—offers significant health benefits without overwhelming their system.

Start by planning your fasts around periods of low stress, ensuring you can focus on rest, hydration, and relaxation. Gradually increase the duration of your fasts as you become more comfortable and experienced. Incorporating shorter fasts, like intermittent fasting (12 to 16 hours of fasting daily), can also serve as a bridge between longer water fasts and daily eating habits.

2. Listening to Your Body: Water fasting is a powerful practice, but it's essential to listen to your body throughout the process. If you feel fatigued, dizzy, or experience any

warning signs, take it as a signal to modify or stop your fast. Your body will communicate what it needs, so being mindful of these signals ensures that water fasting enhances your health rather than depletes it.

Fasting should never feel like punishment or deprivation. Instead, view it as a gift of rest and rejuvenation for your body. Approach it with selfcare in mind, taking the time to engage in meditation, light stretching, or gentle walks to support your wellbeing.

3. Pairing Fasting with a Balanced Lifestyle: To maximize the benefits of water fasting, it should be integrated into a wellrounded lifestyle. This includes regular exercise, a nutritious diet, stress management, and adequate sleep. Fasting helps with detoxification and metabolic reset, but the longterm benefits are only sustained when paired with healthy habits.

After a fast, maintaining balanced eating patterns is crucial. Opt for whole, unprocessed foods that support digestion and provide your body with essential nutrients. Avoid returning to unhealthy habits like overconsumption of processed foods, sugars, or excessive caffeine.

4. Using Fasting for Mental Clarity and Focus: Beyond the physical benefits, water fasting can also help sharpen mental clarity and focus. During fasting, your body enters ketosis, which can boost brain function, enhance cognitive performance, and improve mood. Many individuals report heightened creativity, concentration, and emotional clarity after completing a fast.

Use fasting as an opportunity to reflect on your personal health goals and overall wellness journey. Journaling, meditating, or setting new intentions during this time can provide profound insights and support personal growth.

5. Community and Support: Having a support system can be incredibly beneficial when incorporating water fasting into your wellness routine. Whether it's family, friends, or online fasting communities, sharing your experience can provide encouragement and accountability. Fasting with others can help alleviate any concerns or challenges you may face and also make the process feel more manageable.

5. Periodic Fasting for Long Term Health

Periodic fasting, when done regularly, can significantly contribute to longterm health and longevity. Research shows that fasting can activate powerful cellular repair processes, improve metabolic function, and protect against various chronic diseases. Incorporating periodic fasting into your lifestyle may result in a healthier body, enhanced immune function, and improved energy levels.

1. Benefits of Periodic Fasting: Periodic fasting, such as engaging in a water fast once a month or quarterly, can provide numerous longterm benefits:

Cellular Repair and Autophagy: Fasting activates autophagy, a process where cells remove damaged components and regenerate new, healthier ones. This can help prevent the development of agerelated diseases and promote longevity.

Improved Insulin Sensitivity: Fasting can reduce insulin resistance and help stabilize blood sugar levels, which lowers the risk of type 2 diabetes and other metabolic disorders.

Heart Health: Periodic fasting can improve cholesterol levels, reduce inflammation, and lower blood pressure, which supports cardiovascular health.

Enhanced Brain Health: Fasting has neuroprotective effects, potentially reducing the risk of neurodegenerative diseases like Alzheimer's and Parkinson's by promoting the growth of new brain cells.

2. Hormonal Balance and Weight Management: Fasting influences key hormones related to hunger and metabolism, including insulin, leptin, and ghrelin. By fasting periodically, you give your body a chance to reset its hormone levels, which can help regulate appetite, improve fat metabolism, and support longterm weight management.

Periodic fasting also supports the body's natural circadian rhythm, which is linked to hormone production and metabolic regulation. By allowing your body to rest from constant food intake, fasting can improve the balance of these hormones over time.

3. Implementing a Sustainable Fasting Schedule: Creating a sustainable fasting schedule is crucial to making fasting part

of your longterm health plan. Start by fasting for shorter durations—such as 16 to 24 hours—and slowly increase the length of your fasts. Aim to fast periodically (once a month or quarterly) rather than daily, allowing your body to adjust to these phases of rest and recovery.

Remember that fasting doesn't need to be rigid. If you feel it's necessary, modify your fasting routine to accommodate your lifestyle, physical health, and energy levels. Listening to your body and maintaining flexibility will prevent burnout or negative effects associated with excessive fasting.

4. LongTerm Health Benefits Beyond Fasting: While fasting provides immediate benefits like detoxification, increased energy, and reduced inflammation, its longterm effects extend far beyond the fasting period. By committing to periodic fasting, you're investing in your longterm health, preventing the onset of diseases, and enhancing your body's resilience to environmental stressors.

Incorporating periodic fasting into your wellness journey allows you to unlock these benefits without significantly altering your daily routine. When paired with a balanced lifestyle, fasting can become a powerful tool for maintaining health, vitality, and longevity over the years.

Conclusion: Making water fasting a consistent part of your wellness journey and embracing periodic fasting for longterm health ensures that you're optimizing both your physical and mental wellbeing. Whether for detoxification, mental clarity, or metabolic health, fasting offers powerful benefits when used in conjunction with a holistic approach to lifestyle and nutrition. With a wellplanned fasting routine, you can support your body's natural processes for years to come, fostering lasting health and vitality.

9 798304 002288